An Adult Coloring Book Featuring Funny, Humorous
& Stress Relieving Designs for Sonographers and Ultrasound Techs.

By © Neo coloration

Copyright © Neo Coloration. All rights reserved.
No portion of this publication may be reproduced or transmitted in any form or by any means,
electronic or mechanical, including, but not limited to, audio recording, facsimiles, photocopying,
or information storage and retrieval systems without explicit written permission from the publisher.

Thank you for purchasing this title, we hope you enjoy coloring this book! Neo Coloration is a young start-up dedicated to creating a variety of adult coloring books.

We love what we do and everyday we strive to improve our products to provide you with the best coloring experience. Your feedback is important as well if you have any, don't hesitate to contact us at neocoloration@mail.com

Other titles you may like:
Motivational Swear Word Coloring Book:
Do More of What Makes You F*cking Happy.
(ASIN B083XX25RZ)

Believe in Yourself:
An Adult Coloring Book Featuring Motivational
Sayings and Positive Affirmations.
(ASIN B084DGPN6N)

Without your voice, we don't exist.
Please support us and leave a review!
Thank you!

Coloring can enhance individuation and promote self-discovery.
Focusing on the lines of the pattern helps reduce stress and anxiety, stay present at the moment, easing anxiety about the past and worries about the future. besides getting a dose of humor and laughter that relaxes your whole body and decreases stress hormones etc...

Diagnostic medical sonographers, also known as ultrasound technicians, help doctors, and other health care professionals assess and identify a patient's medical conditions. These professionals use imaging equipment that produces high-frequency waves to record images or conduct tests on many parts of the body.
Sonographers are just superheroes in disguise.

Working as a Sonographer / Ultrasound tech isn't easy and can be very stressful. Relax, have a seat and grab this coloring book it's all what you need, the best stress-relieving activities that help you stay inspired and in the moment. Feel relaxed and melts stress away if you want to continue to function at your best.

This book contains 25 pages of funny and humorous Sonography related designs and sayings surrounded by beautiful artwork, mandalas, and flowers, etc... Relax and enjoy some good vibes that will level up your confidence and will give you encouragement throughout the daily stress of life.

- Black background reverse pages to reduce bleed-through
- Each page is single-sided for getting the best coloring experience

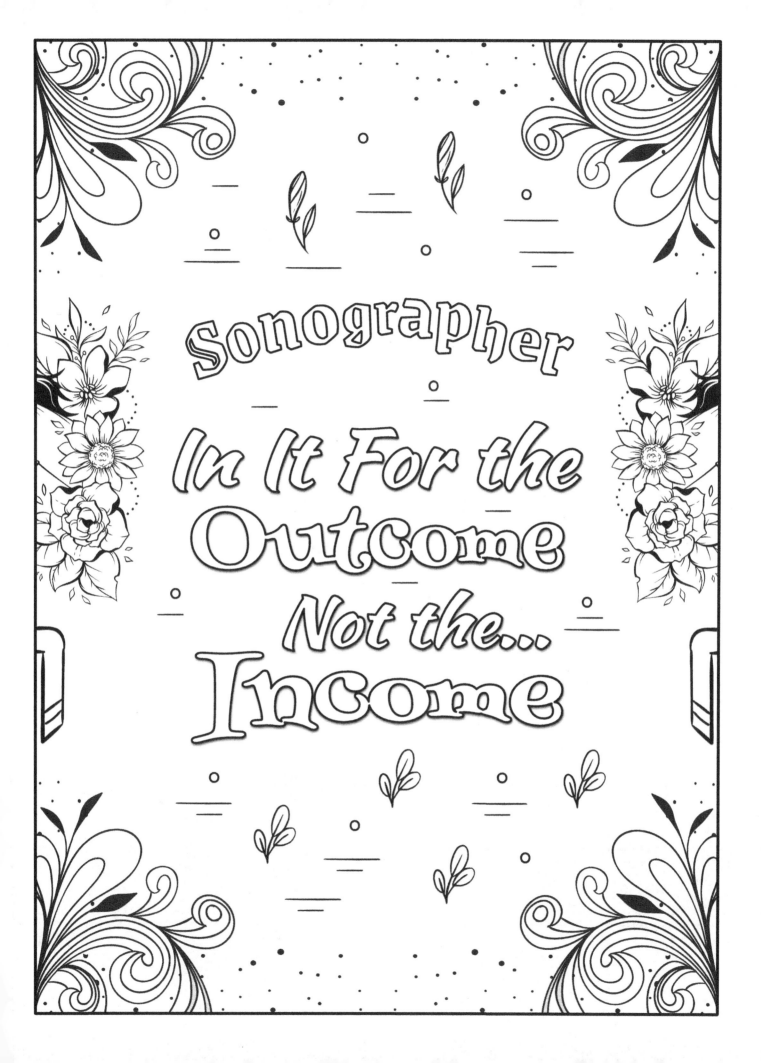

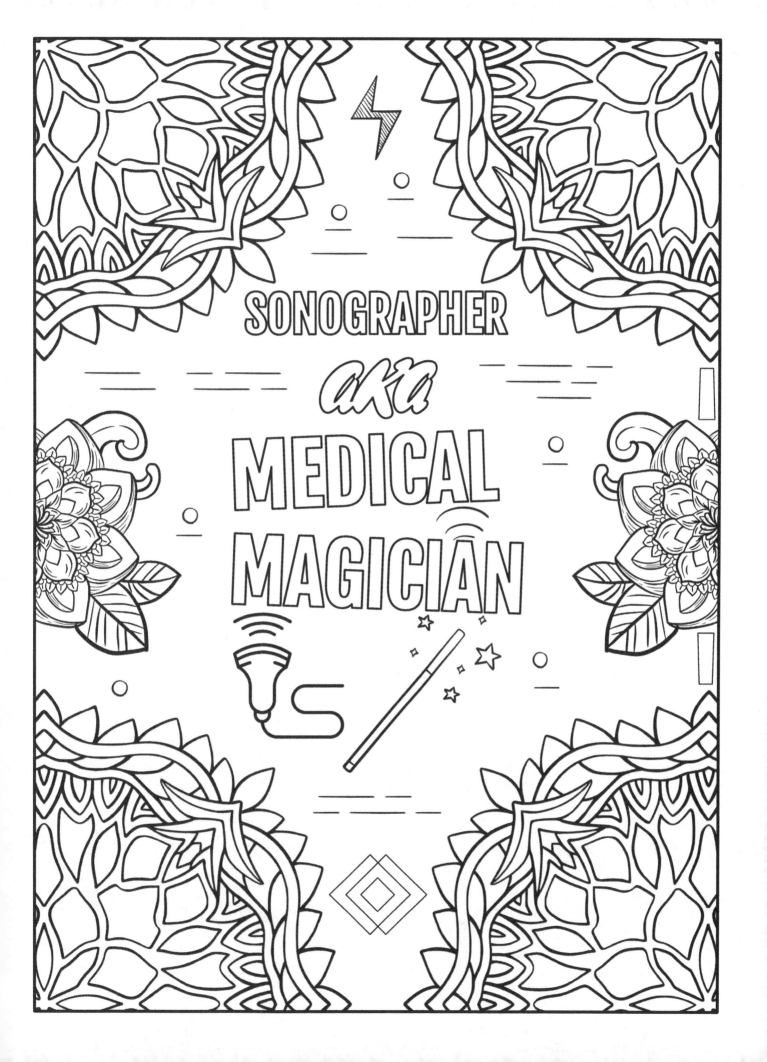

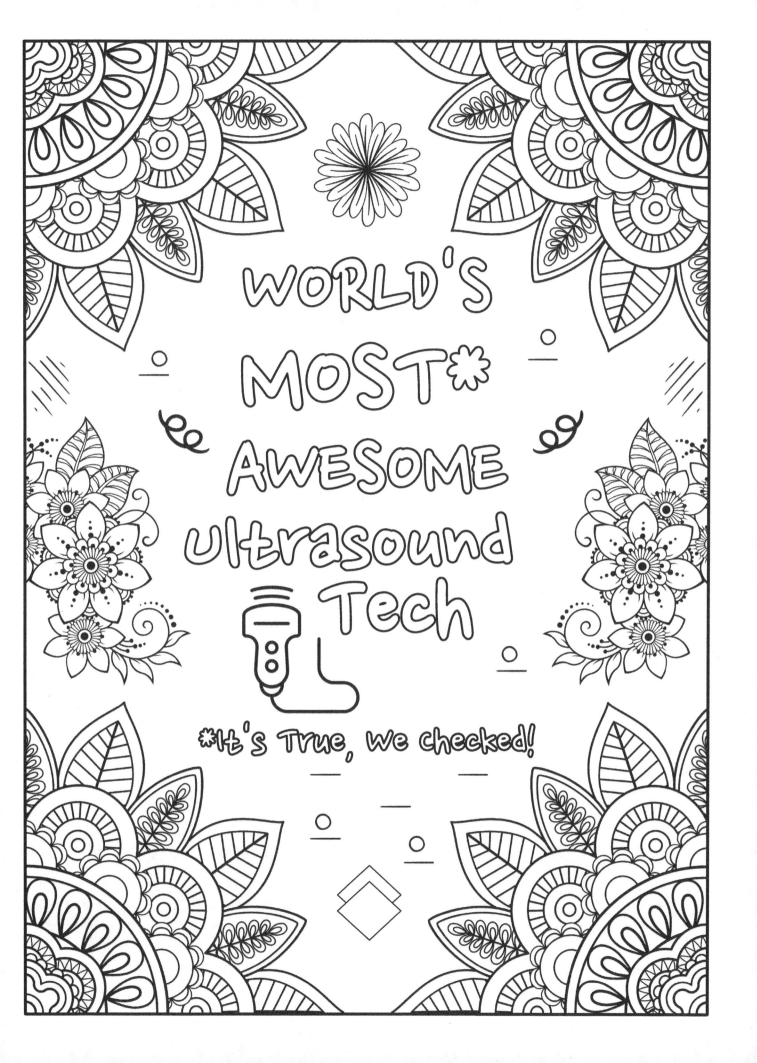

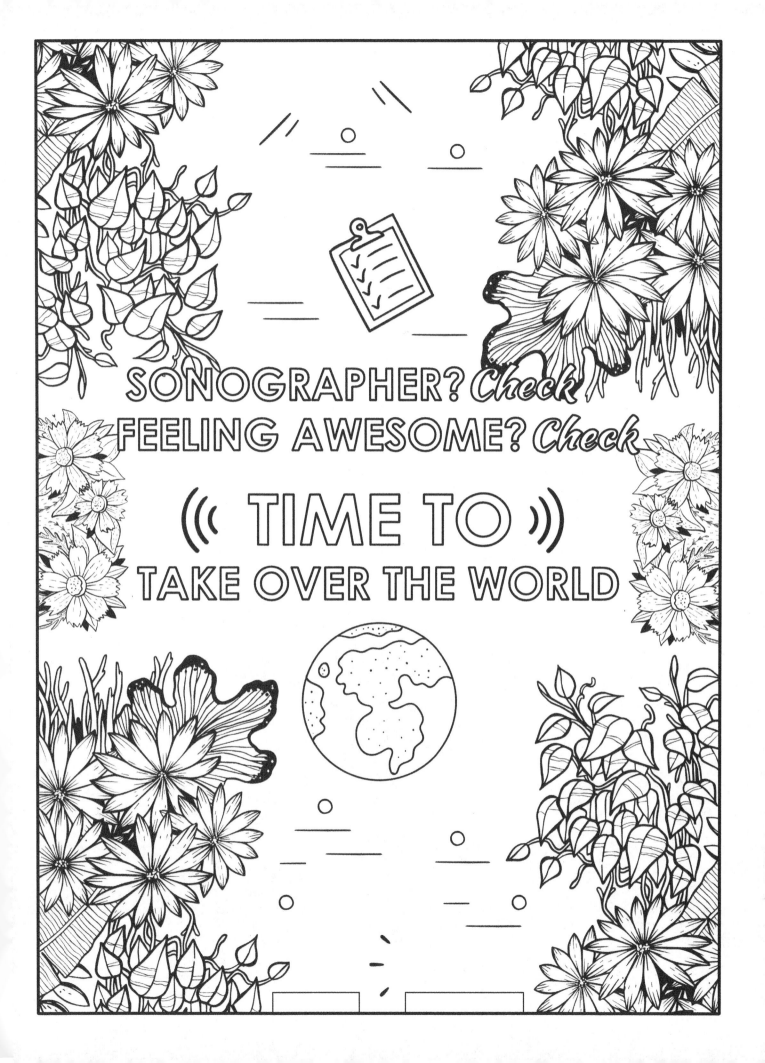

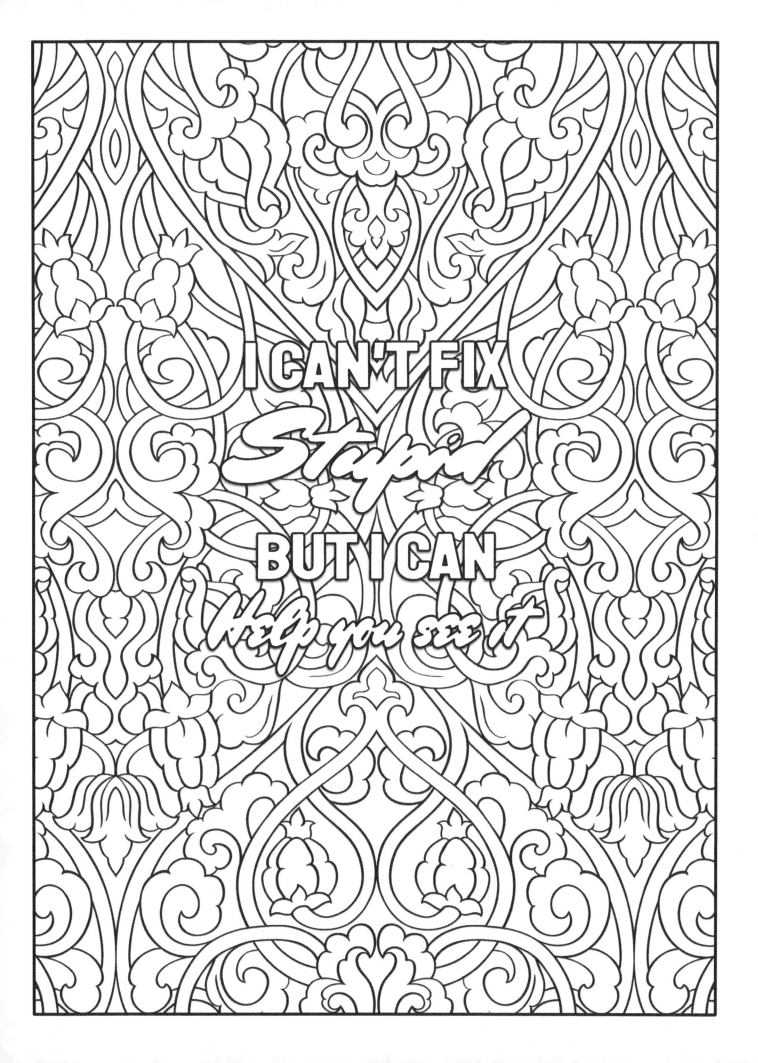

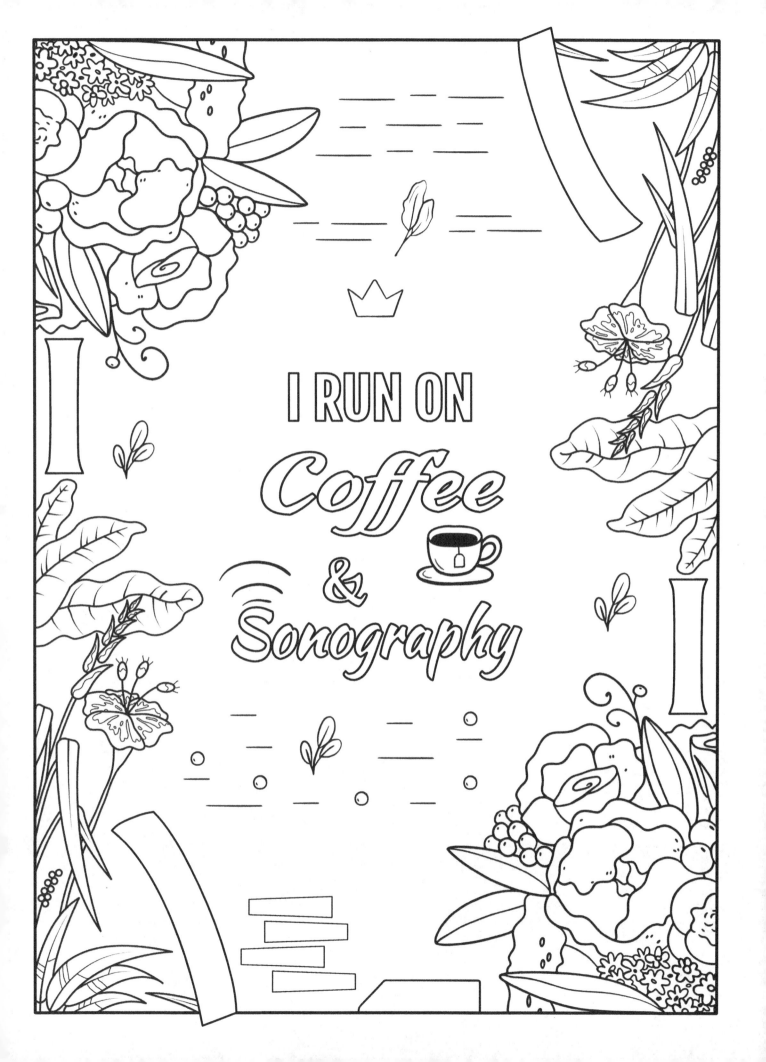

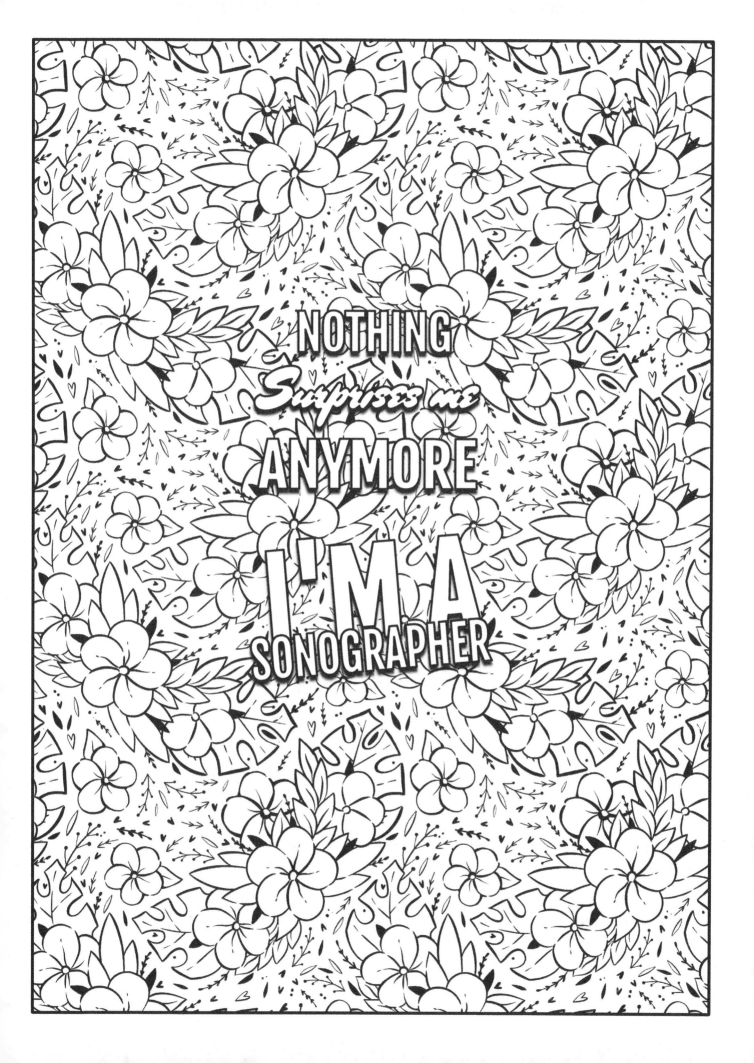

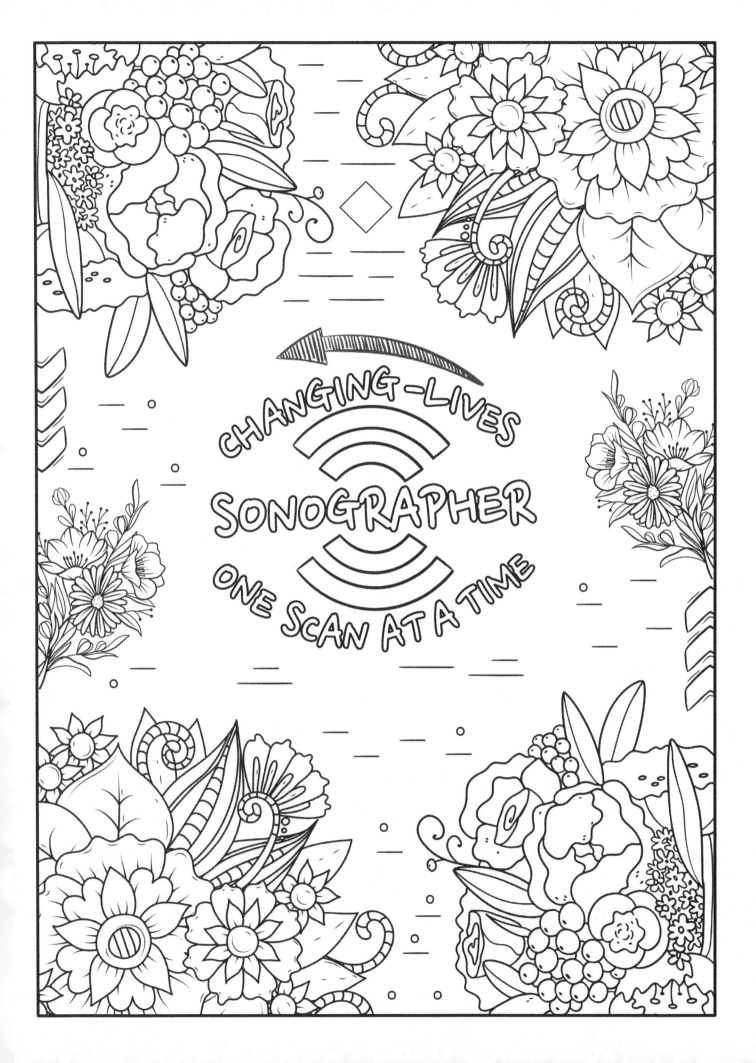

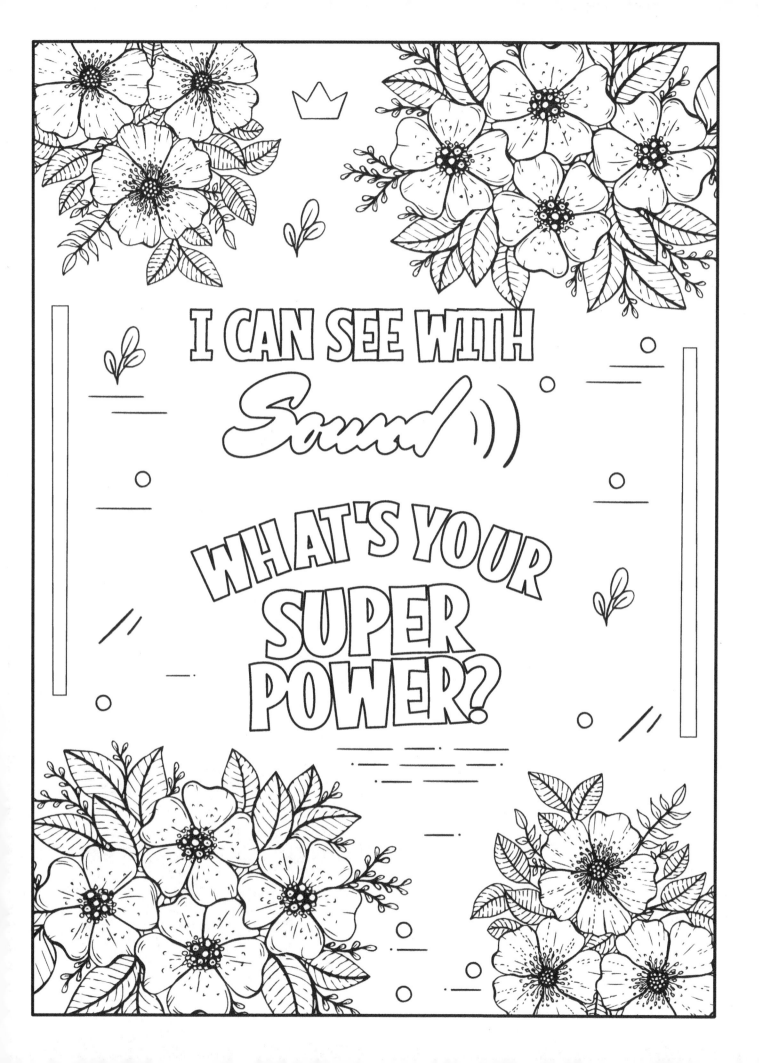

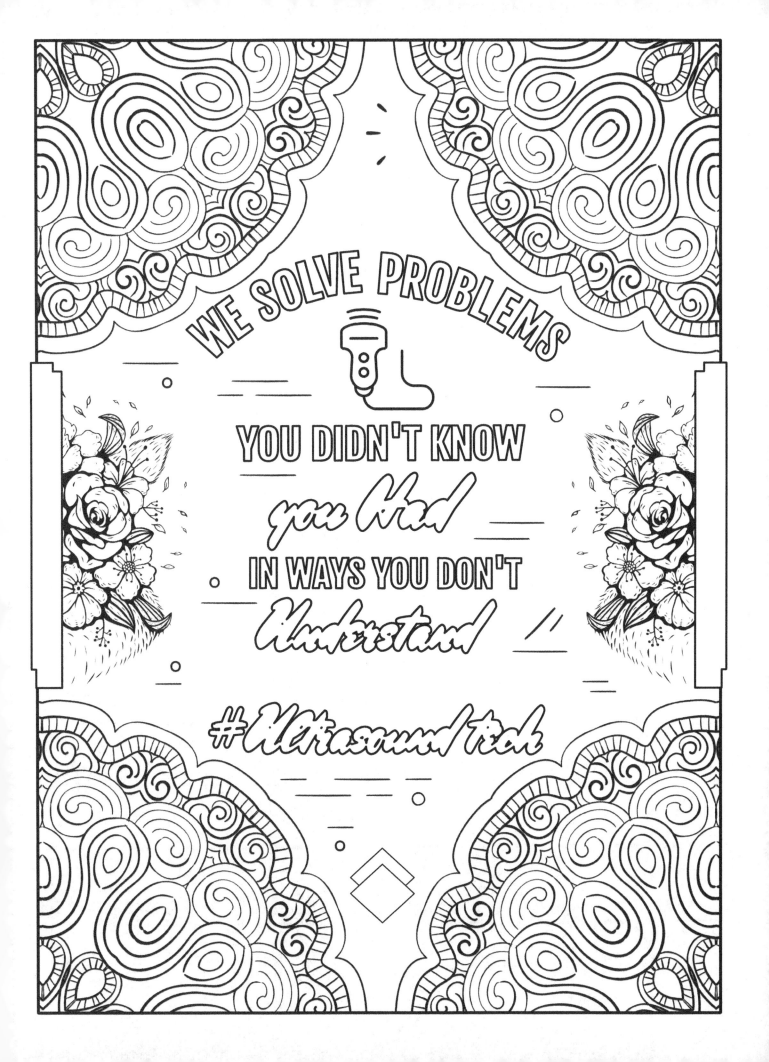

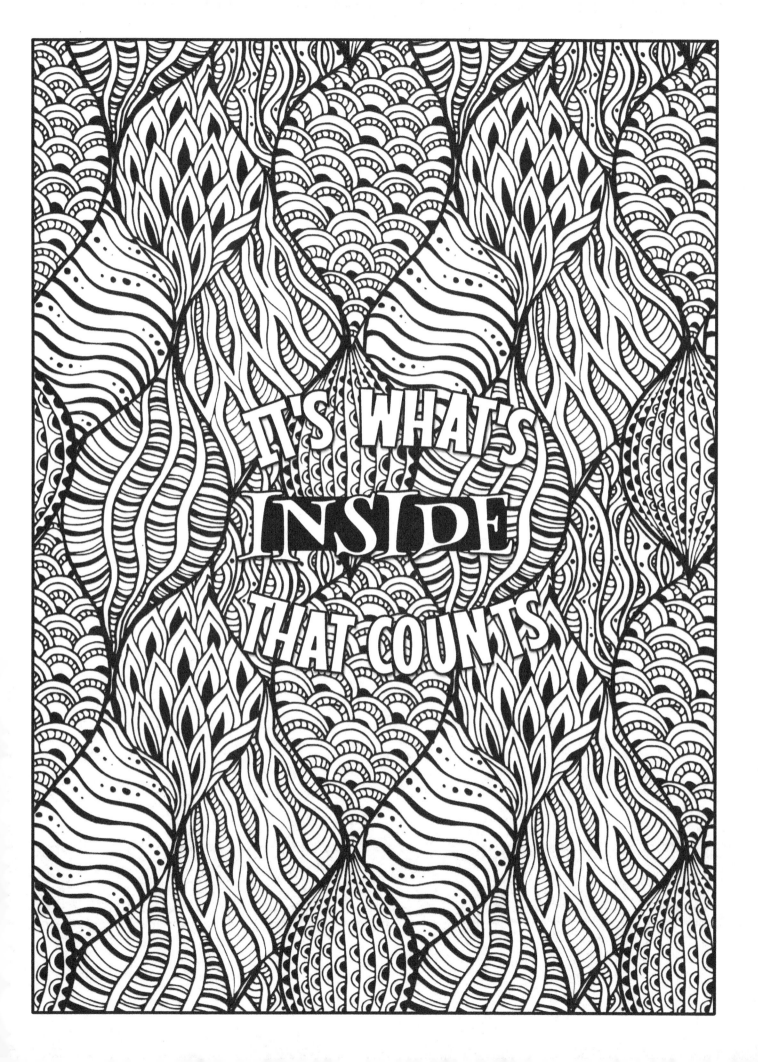

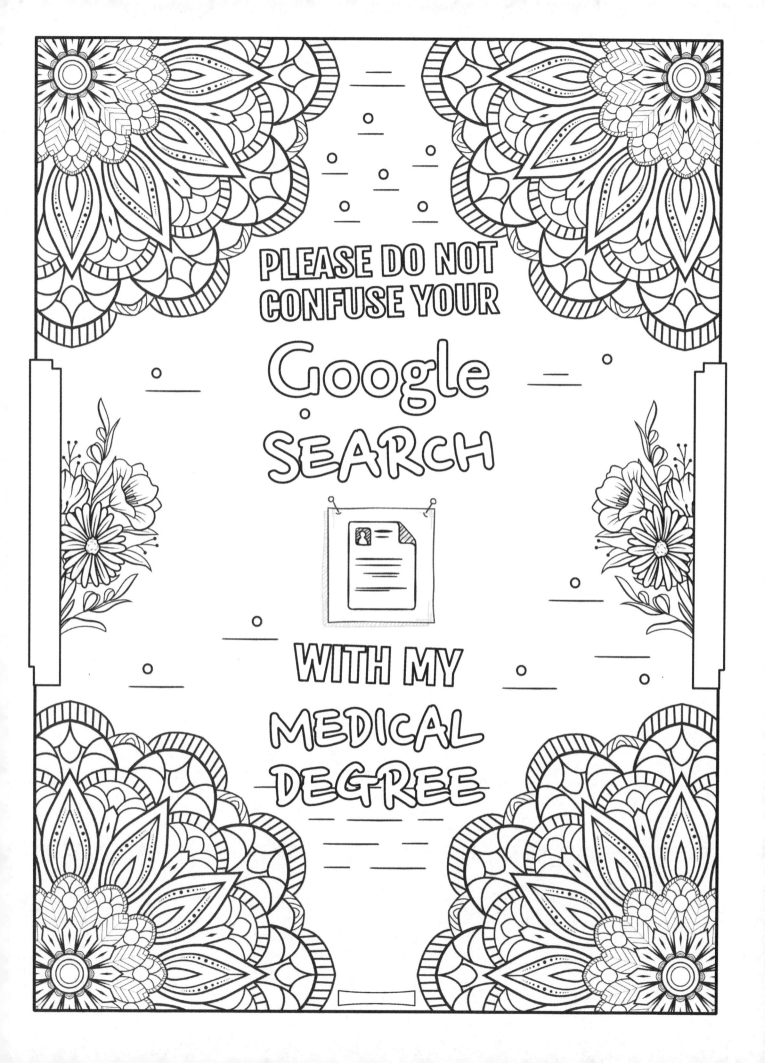

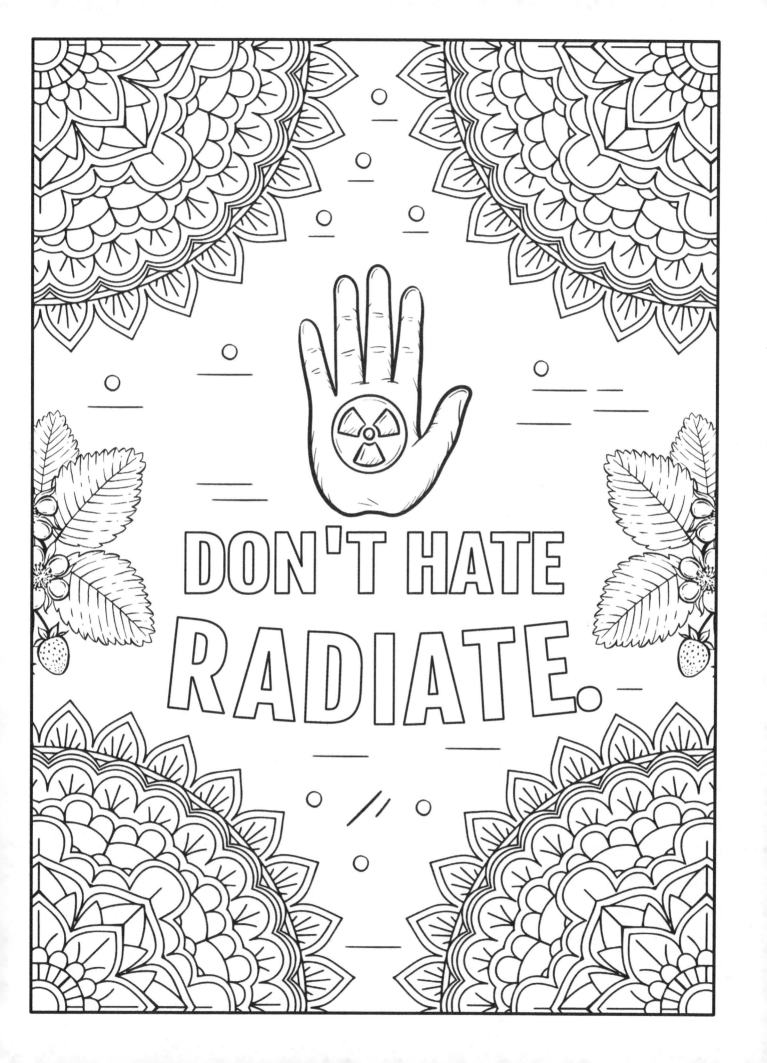

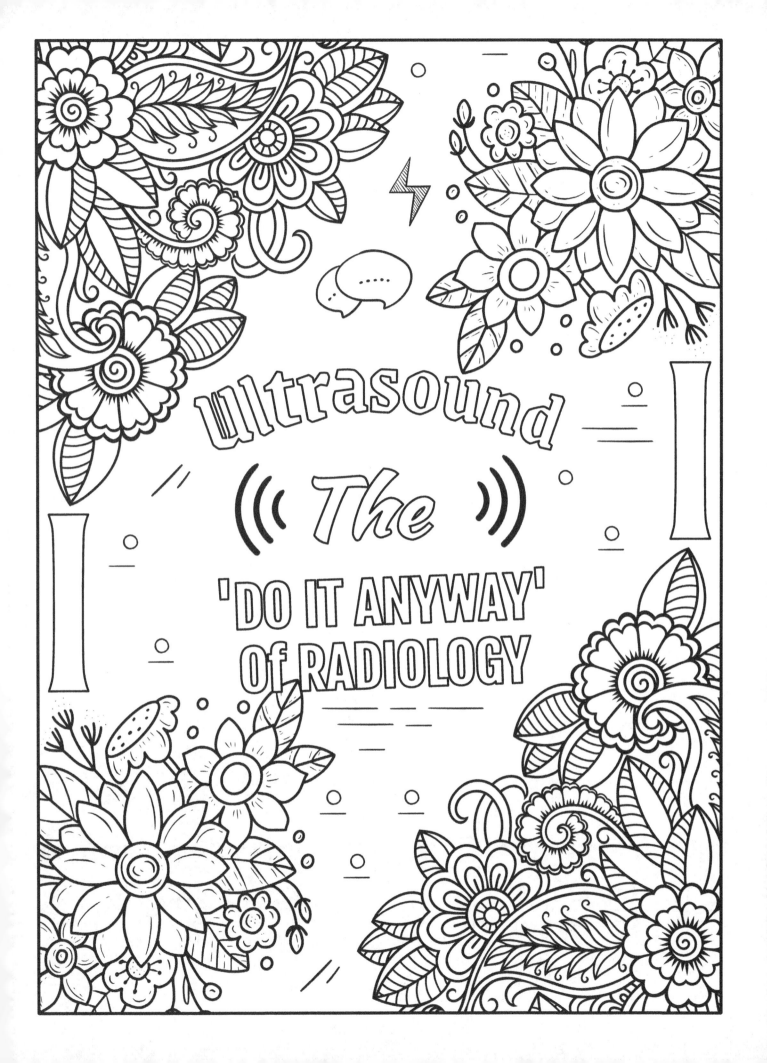

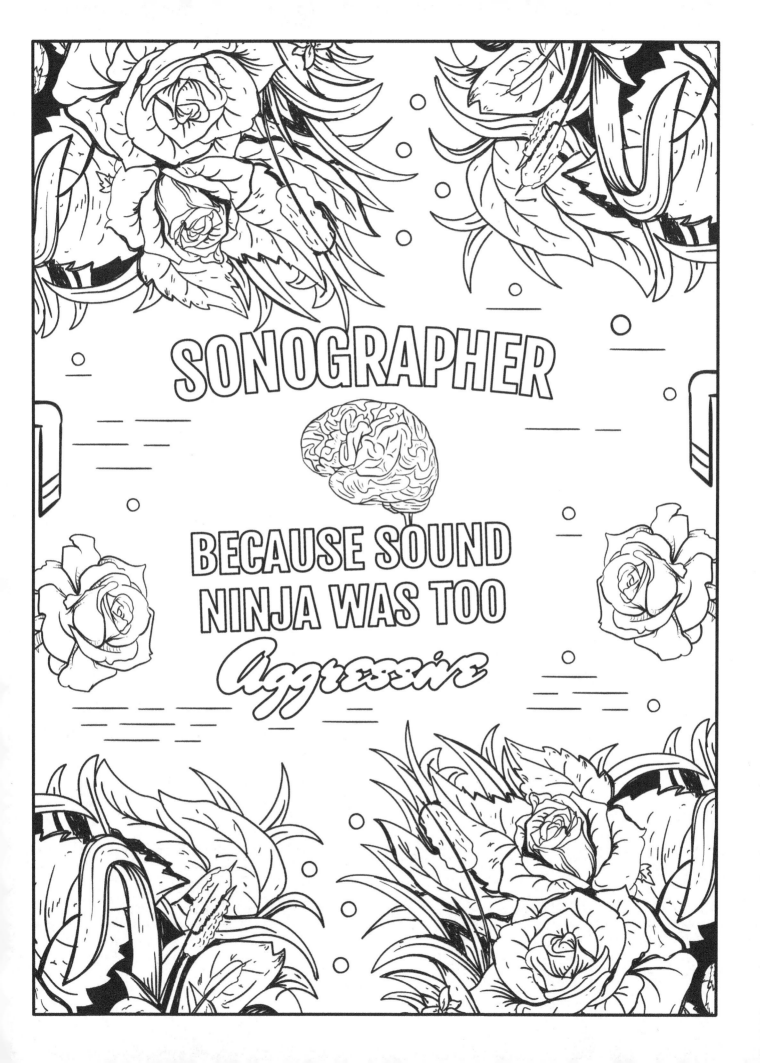

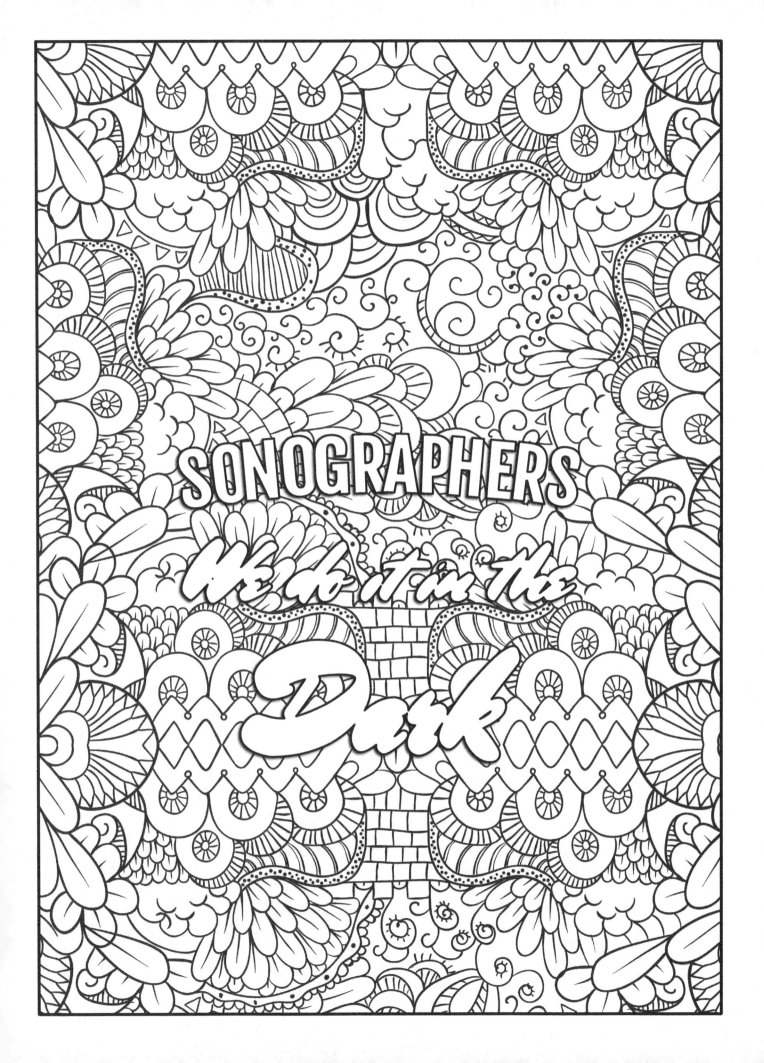

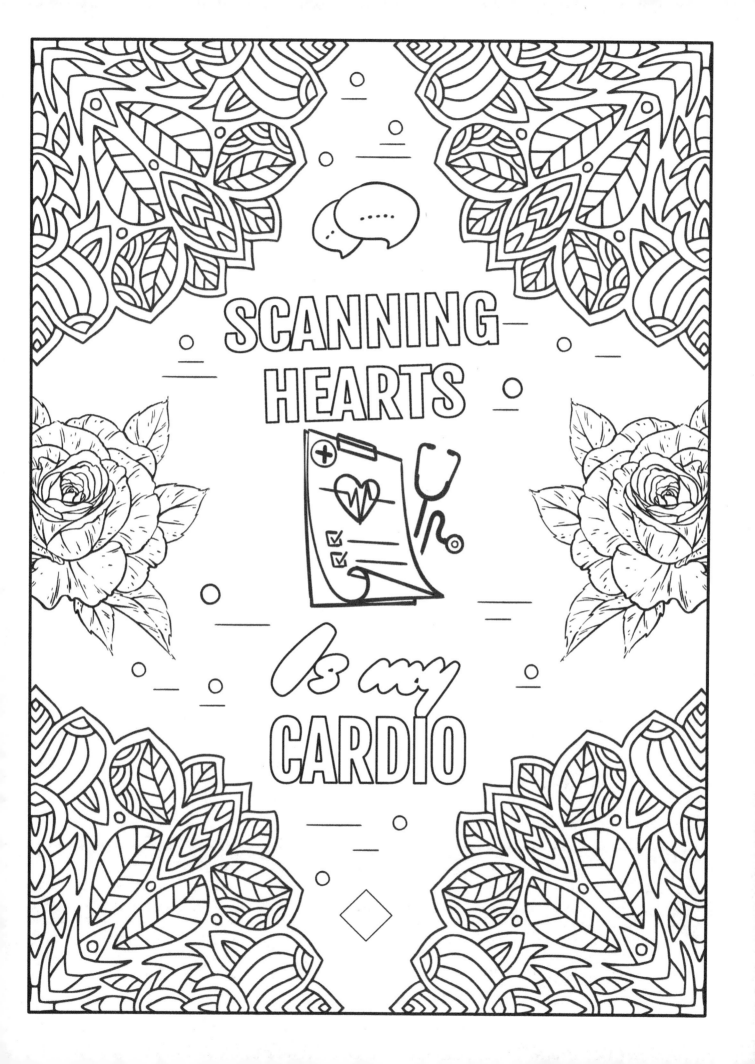

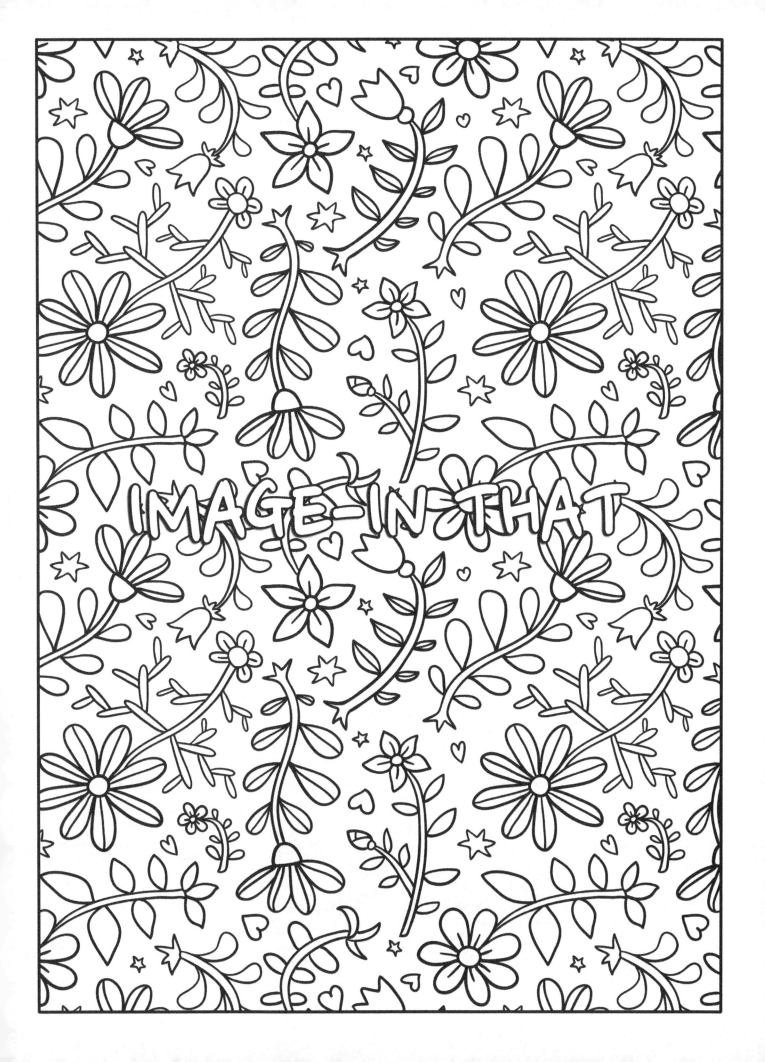

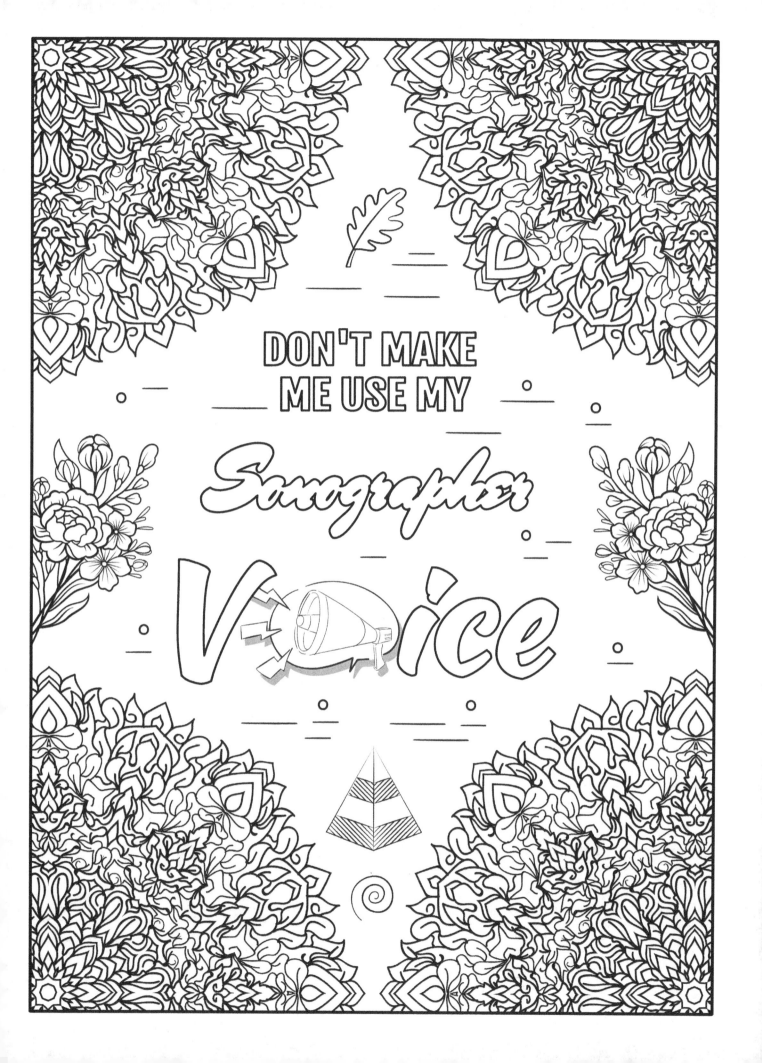

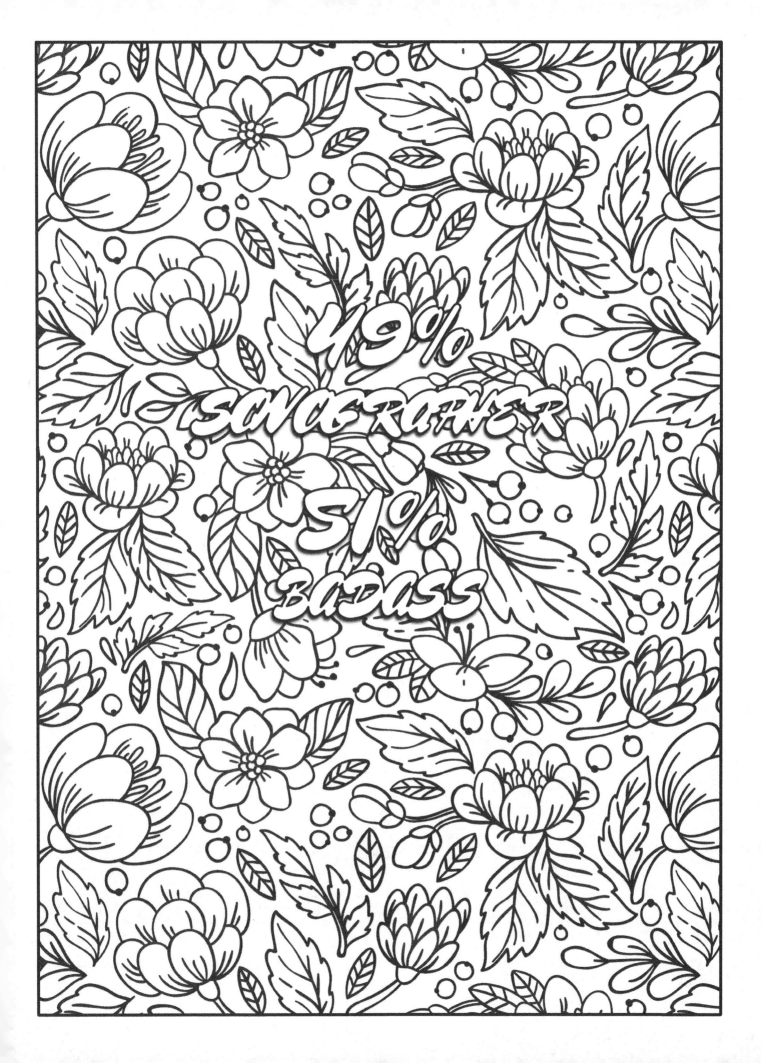

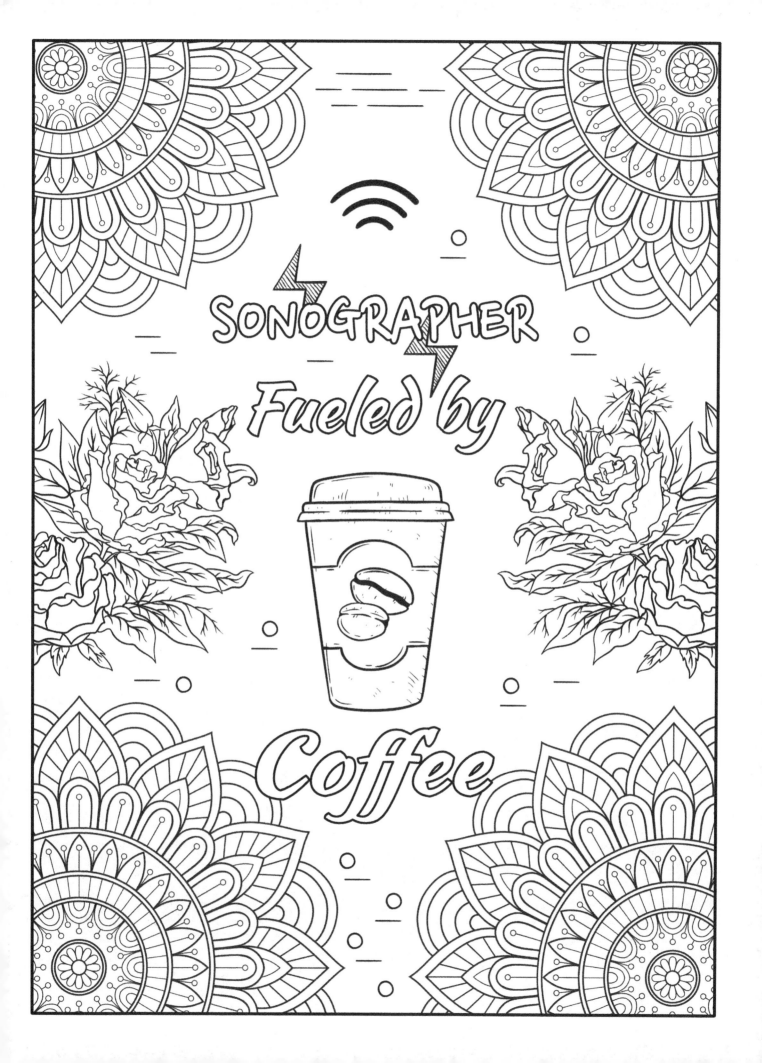

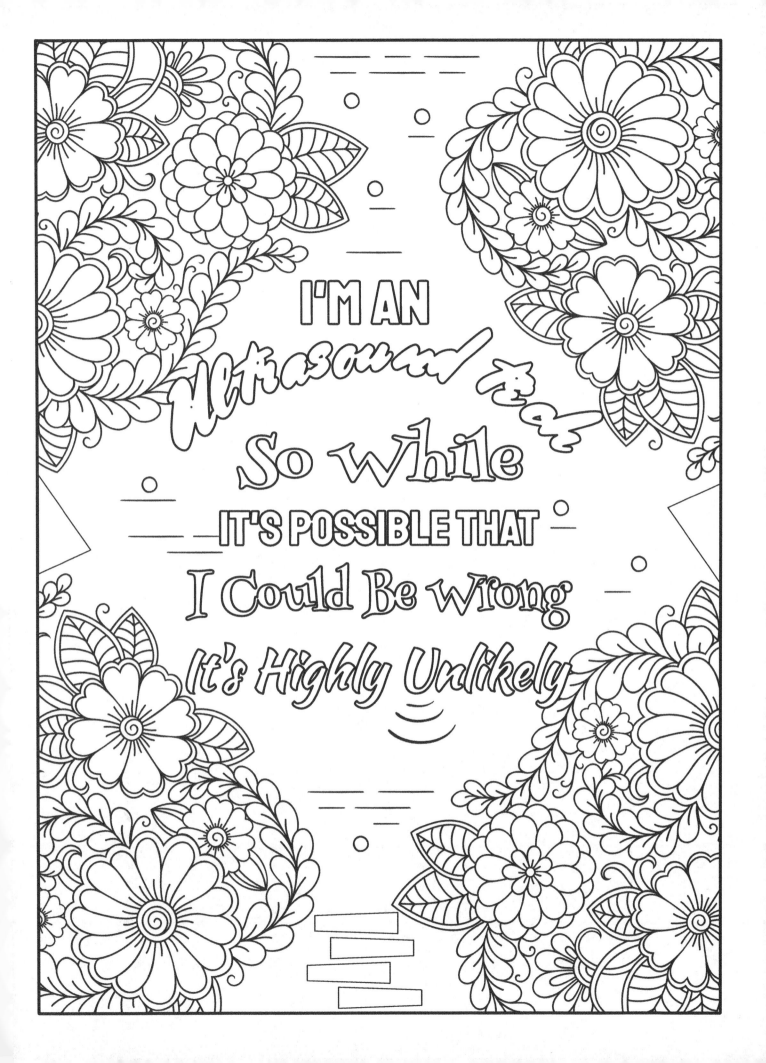

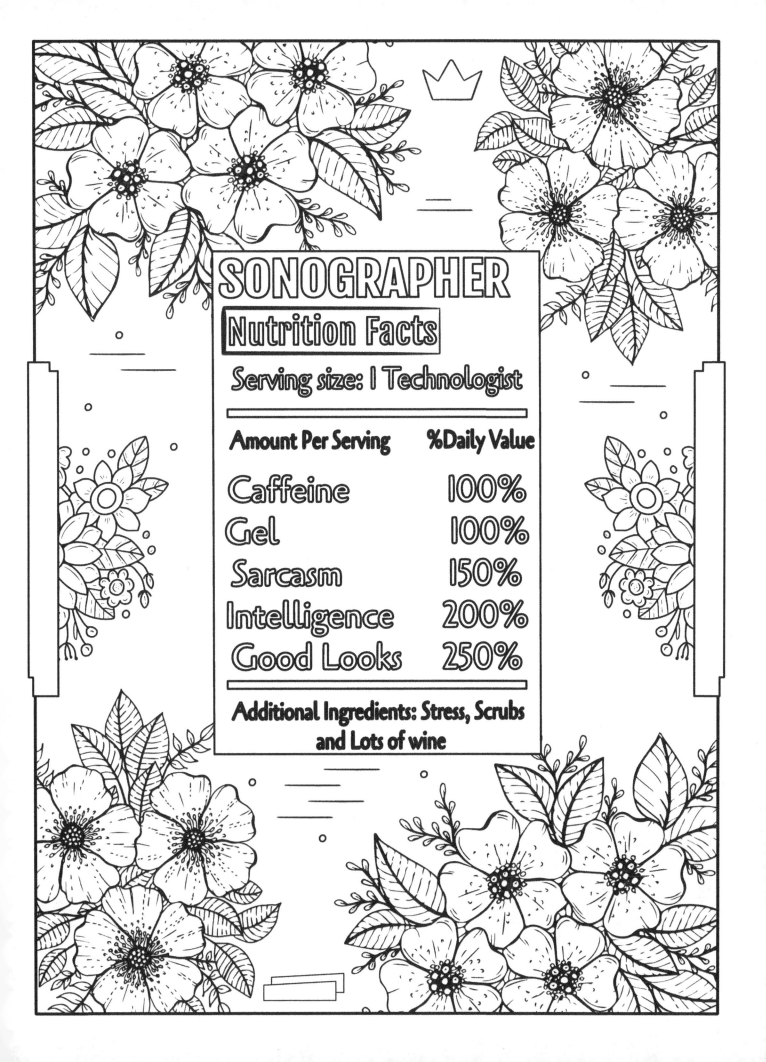

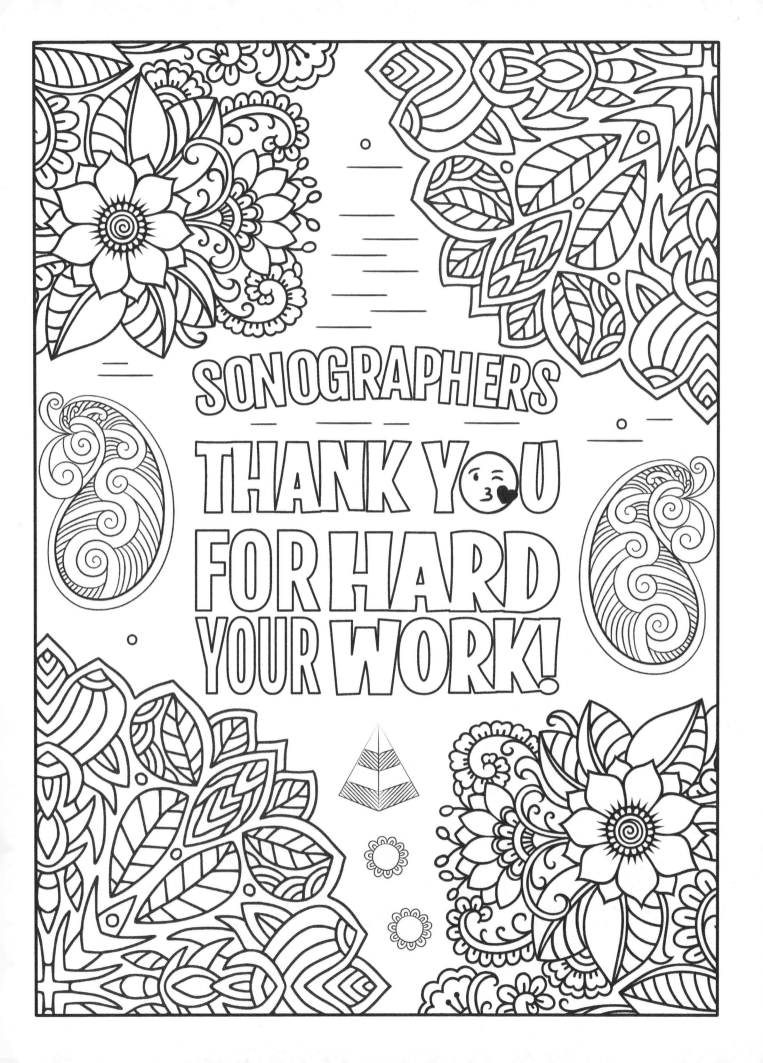

# Color test page

## Color test page

Made in United States
North Haven, CT
18 December 2024

63082100R00037